# COMPREHENSIVE PAIN MANAGEMENT

*A Guide for Medical Doctors*

Dr Essam Abdelhakim

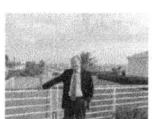

Copyright © 2024 Dr Essam Abdelhakim

All rights reserved

The characters and events portrayed in this book are fictitious. Any similarity to real persons, living or dead, is coincidental and not intended by the author.

No part of this book may be reproduced, or stored in a retrieval system, or transmitted in any form or by any means, electronic, mechanical, photocopying, recording, or otherwise, without express written permission of the publisher.

Cover design by: Art Painter
Library of Congress Control Number: 2018675309
Printed in the United States of America

# CONTENTS

Title Page
Copyright
Introduction
Chapter 1: Introduction to Pain Management — 1
Chapter 2: Assessment and Diagnosis of Pain — 5
Chapter 3: Pharmacological Approaches to Pain Management — 10
Chapter 4: Non-Pharmacological Therapies for Pain Management — 16
Chapter 5: Interventional Pain Management Techniques — 21
Chapter 6: Surgical Approaches to Pain Management — 26
Chapter 7: Chronic Pain Management Strategies — 31
Chapter 8: Pediatric Pain Management — 36
Chapter 9: Geriatric Pain Management — 40
Chapter 10: Pain Management in Special Populations — 44
Chapter 11: Regulatory and Ethical Considerations — 50
Chapter 12: Emerging Trends and Future Directions in Pain Management — 57
Chapter 13: 20 Case Studies and Clinical Scenarios — 63
About The Author — 85
Disclosure — 87

# INTRODUCTION

*Pain is one of the most common and challenging conditions encountered by medical practitioners across all specialties.*

*Whether acute or chronic, pain has a profound impact on a patiens quality of life, and its management remains a cornerstone of medical practice.*
*Effective pain management requires an in-depth understanding of its multifaceted nature, the various therapeutic options available, and the ability to tailor these approaches to individual patients.*

**This book,** *Comprehensive Pain Management: A Guide for Medical Doctors*, aims to provide healthcare professionals with the knowledge and tools necessary to assess, diagnose, and treat pain effectively.

*It addresses a broad spectrum of pain management strategies, from pharmacological interventions to non-pharmacological and interventional techniques, ensuring that clinicians can apply a holistic approach to pain treatment.*

**The book** is structured to cover key areas in pain management, beginning with an understanding of the complex physiology of pain and moving through essential topics such as pharmacological approaches, non-pharmacological therapies, interventional treatments, surgical strategies, and specialized approaches for managing pain in specific populations.

Each chapter provides practical insights, evidence-based practices, and real-world clinical scenarios to guide clinicians in making informed decisions for optimal patient outcomes.

# CHAPTER 1: INTRODUCTION TO PAIN MANAGEMENT

### 1.1 Definition of Pain and Types

*Pain is a complex, multidimensional experience that encompasses sensory, emotional, and cognitive components.*

*The International Association for the Study of Pain (IASP) defines pain as "an unpleasant sensory and emotional experience associated with, or resembling that associated with, actual or potential tissue damage."*

*This broad definition recognizes that pain is subjective, influenced by numerous factors, and is far more than a mere physical sensation.*

## Types Of Pain:

- **Acute Pain**: This type of pain typically has a sudden onset and is directly related to tissue damage, such as injury, surgery, or infection. Acute pain serves as a protective mechanism that alerts the body to potential harm and typically resolves once the underlying cause has healed.
- **Chronic Pain**: Defined as pain that persists for more than three months or beyond the expected period of healing. Unlike acute pain, chronic pain may not have a clear cause and can persist even after tissue damage has healed. Chronic pain often leads to significant psychological, emotional, and functional impairments.
- **Nociceptive Pain**: This pain arises from the activation

of nociceptors, which are sensory receptors that detect harmful stimuli. It is typically subdivided into **somatic** pain (originating from skin, muscles, and joints) and **visceral** pain (arising from internal organs).

- **Neuropathic Pain**: Caused by injury or dysfunction of the nervous system, neuropathic pain often presents as burning, tingling, or shooting sensations. Common causes include diabetic neuropathy, nerve trauma, and postherpetic neuralgia.
- **Mixed Pain Syndromes**: Certain pain conditions involve a combination of nociceptive and neuropathic pain components, such as complex regional pain syndrome (CRPS) and some cancer-related pains.

## 1.2 The Physiology Of Pain

Understanding the physiological mechanisms underlying pain is crucial for effective management.

The perception of pain involves a complex series of steps that can be broadly categorized as:

- **Transduction**: This is the process by which noxious stimuli, such as thermal, mechanical, or chemical stimuli, are converted into electrical signals by nociceptors.
- **Transmission**: Once transduced, these electrical signals are transmitted via peripheral nerves to the spinal cord and brain. The signals travel through various pathways, such as the spinothalamic tract, which relays sensory information to the brain for processing.
- **Perception**: This refers to the conscious awareness and interpretation of pain. It occurs in higher brain centers, including the thalamus, somatosensory cortex, limbic system, and prefrontal cortex. Perception involves not

only recognizing the sensation but also associating emotional and cognitive dimensions.
- **Modulation**: This step involves the regulation of pain signals by endogenous inhibitory pathways, such as the descending pain-modulating system. Neurotransmitters like endorphins and enkephalins can inhibit pain signals, while conditions like stress, anxiety, and depression can exacerbate them.

## 1.3 The Biopsychosocial Model Of Pain

Modern pain management approaches emphasize a biopsychosocial model, recognizing that pain is not merely a physical experience but a complex interplay of biological, psychological, and social factors.

This model provides a more holistic understanding of how pain impacts patients and underscores the importance of a comprehensive approach to treatment.

**Biological Factors:**
- Tissue damage and nociceptive activation
- Genetic predisposition to pain sensitivity or chronic pain syndromes
- Neurological dysfunction, such as nerve injury

**Psychological Factors:**
- Emotions, such as fear, anxiety, and depression
- Coping mechanisms and individual resilience
- Catastrophizing and negative thought patterns

**Social Factors:**
- Support systems and family dynamics
- Socioeconomic status and access to healthcare
- Cultural attitudes and beliefs about pain and pain management

## 1.4 Importance Of Multidisciplinary Pain Management

Given the multifaceted nature of pain, effective management often requires a multidisciplinary approach that combines expertise from various healthcare professionals, including physicians, psychologists, physical therapists, pharmacists, and others.

This collaborative approach ensures that the biological, psychological, and social aspects of pain are addressed, leading to better patient outcomes.

### Benefits Of A Multidisciplinary Approach:

- Comprehensive assessment and tailored treatment plans
- Reduced reliance on opioids and pharmacological interventions alone
- Enhanced patient education and self-management strategies
- Improved quality of life and functional restoration

# CHAPTER 2: ASSESSMENT AND DIAGNOSIS OF PAIN

## 2.1 Clinical History And Physical Examination

*Effective pain management begins with a thorough and detailed assessment.*

*An accurate diagnosis is critical to understanding the underlying cause of pain and tailoring appropriate management strategies.*

*The foundation of assessment includes a comprehensive clinical history and physical examination.*

**Clinical History** *A detailed history helps to characterize the pain and can provide vital clues about its etiology and contributing factors.*

*Key elements of the history include:*

- **Onset and Duration**: Understanding whether the pain is acute, subacute, or chronic.
- **Location and Radiation**: The precise location of the pain and whether it radiates to other regions.
- **Quality**: Description of the pain (e.g., sharp, dull, burning, throbbing, aching).
- **Intensity**: Assessment of pain severity, often quantified using pain scales.
- **Aggravating and Alleviating Factors**: Identifying factors that worsen or improve the pain.
- **Associated Symptoms**: Symptoms such as numbness, weakness, swelling, or systemic symptoms (e.g., fever, weight loss).

- **Impact on Function**: The effect of pain on daily activities, sleep, work, and quality of life.
- **Medical, Surgical, and Family History**: Relevant history, including past treatments for pain and family predisposition to certain conditions.
- **Psychosocial History**: Stress, anxiety, depression, or substance use history, which may influence pain perception and response to treatment.

**Physical Examination**

*A thorough physical examination helps to localize the pain source, assess functional impairment, and identify signs suggestive of specific conditions.*

*Key components include:*

- **Inspection**: Observation for signs of injury, deformity, swelling, discoloration, or muscle wasting.
- **Palpation**: Gentle pressure applied to assess tenderness, tissue texture, or the presence of masses.
- **Range of Motion (ROM)**: Evaluation of joint mobility and flexibility, noting any restrictions or pain during movement.
- **Neurological Examination**: Assessment of reflexes, muscle strength, sensory deficits, and nerve function.
- **Special Tests**: Depending on the suspected condition, special maneuvers or tests (e.g., straight leg raise test for sciatica) may be performed.

## 2.2 Pain Scales And Assessment Tools

*Quantifying pain is essential for monitoring treatment progress and tailoring interventions.*

*Several standardized pain assessment tools are used in clinical practice:*

## Common Pain Scales:

- **Numeric Rating Scale (NRS)**: Patients rate their pain on a scale from 0 (no pain) to 10 (worst pain imaginable).
- **Visual Analog Scale (VAS)**: A 10-centimeter line where patients mark their pain level, providing a continuous measure of pain intensity.
- **Verbal Rating Scale (VRS)**: Patients describe their pain as none, mild, moderate, or severe.
- **Faces Pain Scale**: Often used for pediatric or non-verbal patients, featuring faces depicting different levels of pain.

## Specialized Assessment Tools:

- **McGill Pain Questionnaire**: Assesses qualitative aspects of pain using descriptive terms and sensory, affective, and evaluative categories.
- **Brief Pain Inventory (BPI)**: Measures pain intensity, interference with daily activities, and the impact on function.
- **Pain Disability Index (PDI)**: Assesses the degree to which chronic pain impacts daily life activities, such as work, social interactions, and recreation.

## 2.3 Diagnostic Imaging And Laboratory Tests

*Imaging and laboratory tests are often used to confirm the cause of pain, rule out serious underlying conditions, and guide treatment decisions.*

*However, they should be used judiciously to avoid over-reliance, especially in cases where structural findings may not correlate with the severity of pain.*

**Common Diagnostic Imaging:**
- **X-Rays**: Useful for identifying fractures, joint degeneration, and alignment issues.
- **Magnetic Resonance Imaging (MRI)**: Provides detailed images of soft tissues, including muscles, ligaments, intervertebral discs, and nerve roots. Commonly used in the evaluation of spinal disorders and soft tissue injuries.
- **Computed Tomography (CT)**: Offers cross-sectional views of bones and soft tissues, useful for complex fractures or bone lesions.
- **Ultrasound**: A cost-effective tool for evaluating soft tissue injuries, inflammation, or fluid collections.

**Laboratory Tests:**
- **Inflammatory Markers**: Elevated levels of C-reactive protein (CRP) or erythrocyte sedimentation rate (ESR) may indicate an inflammatory or autoimmune condition.
- **Autoantibodies and Rheumatological Markers**: Tests for rheumatoid factor (RF), anti-nuclear antibodies (ANA), and anti-cyclic citrullinated peptides (anti-CCP) help diagnose autoimmune causes of pain.
- **Infection Screening**: Blood cultures or targeted testing for infectious agents if an infectious cause is suspected.

**2.4 Psychological Assessment and Co-occurring Disorders**

*Psychological factors can significantly influence pain perception, coping mechanisms, and the success of treatment interventions.*

*Addressing co-occurring psychological disorders is essential for effective pain management.*

# Common Psychological Assessments:

- **Depression and Anxiety Scales**: Tools such as the Patient Health Questionnaire-9 (PHQ-9) for depression and the Generalized Anxiety Disorder-7 (GAD-7) scale help identify underlying psychological conditions.
- **Pain Catastrophizing Scale (PCS)**: Evaluates negative thought patterns and the extent to which a patient magnifies the impact of pain.
- **Cognitive and Behavioral Assessments**: Assessments to evaluate how patients think about and cope with their pain, which can guide cognitive-behavioral therapy (CBT) interventions.

## Managing Co-Occurring Disorders:

- **Psychiatric Referrals**: For conditions like depression, anxiety, or post-traumatic stress disorder (PTSD), collaboration with a psychiatrist or psychologist is often necessary.
- **Integrated Behavioral Interventions**: Cognitive-behavioral therapy (CBT), mindfulness-based stress reduction (MBSR), and biofeedback are effective in reducing the psychological burden of chronic pain.

# CHAPTER 3: PHARMACOLOGICAL APPROACHES TO PAIN MANAGEMENT

## 3.1 Non-Opioid Analgesics (Nsaids, Acetaminophen)

**Non-opioid analgesics** *are typically considered as first-line agents in the management of mild to moderate pain and form the cornerstone of pain therapy.*

*They provide effective analgesia for various pain conditions with relatively low risk of dependency.*

**Non-Steroidal Anti-Inflammatory Drugs (NSAIDs)**
- **Mechanism of Action**: NSAIDs inhibit cyclooxygenase (COX) enzymes, thereby reducing the synthesis of prostaglandins that mediate inflammation and pain.
- **Common Examples**: Ibuprofen, naproxen, diclofenac, celecoxib.
- **Indications**: Used for acute pain (e.g., musculoskeletal injuries), chronic inflammatory conditions (e.g., rheumatoid arthritis), and postoperative pain.
- **Benefits**: Anti-inflammatory, analgesic, and antipyretic effects.
- **Risks and Adverse Effects**:
    - **Gastrointestinal (GI) Toxicity**: NSAIDs can cause gastritis, ulcers, and GI bleeding. Use of proton pump inhibitors (PPIs) may be

recommended for patients at risk of GI complications.
- **Renal Impairment**: Prolonged use can impair renal function, particularly in patients with preexisting kidney disease or dehydration.
- **Cardiovascular Risks**: Some NSAIDs, particularly COX-2 inhibitors, have been associated with an increased risk of thrombotic events such as myocardial infarction.

**Acetaminophen (Paracetamol)**
- **Mechanism of Action**: The exact mechanism is not fully understood, but acetaminophen primarily acts centrally, with analgesic and antipyretic effects, but minimal anti-inflammatory activity.
- **Indications**: Commonly used for mild to moderate pain and fever. It is often recommended for osteoarthritis, headaches, and musculoskeletal pain.
- **Benefits**: Low risk of GI and cardiovascular adverse effects, making it a safer option for long-term use in many patients.
- **Risks**: High doses or chronic use can lead to hepatotoxicity. The maximum recommended daily dose should not exceed 4 grams for adults, with caution in patients with liver disease or chronic alcohol use.

## 3.2 Opioid Analgesics: Indications, Benefits, And Risks

**Opioids** are potent analgesics used for moderate to severe pain that is not adequately controlled by non-opioid agents. Their use requires careful consideration due to their significant risks and potential for misuse.

**Mechanism of Action**: Opioids bind to specific receptors in the central and peripheral nervous systems (mu, delta, and kappa receptors), modulating pain perception and response.

**Common Examples**:
- **Weak Opioids**: Codeine, tramadol.
- **Strong Opioids**: Morphine, oxycodone, fentanyl, hydromorphone.

**Indications**:
- **Acute Pain**: Short-term use for severe pain (e.g., postoperative, trauma).
- **Chronic Pain**: Reserved for severe cases of chronic non-cancer pain when other therapies fail and for palliative care settings.
- **Cancer Pain**: Often used as part of a comprehensive approach to manage cancer-related pain.

**Benefits**:
- Effective relief for severe, intractable pain.
- Can improve function and quality of life in carefully selected patients.

**Risks and Adverse Effects**:
- **Respiratory Depression**: The most serious side effect, particularly in opioid-naïve patients or when combined with other CNS depressants.
- **Constipation**: A common side effect due to opioid

effects on the GI tract, requiring prophylactic laxatives.
- **Nausea, Vomiting, and Sedation**: Common early side effects that may decrease with tolerance.
- **Addiction and Dependence**: Long-term use can lead to physical dependence, tolerance, and in some cases, opioid use disorder. Risk mitigation strategies include patient education, careful selection, and monitoring of therapy.

**Considerations for Safe Use:**
- **Start Low and Go Slow**: Especially in opioid-naïve patients or those with significant comorbidities.
- **Opioid Contracts and Monitoring**: Agreements outlining safe opioid use and regular follow-ups, including prescription monitoring program checks, can reduce misuse risks.

## 3.3 Adjuvant Medications (Anticonvulsants, Antidepressants)

*Adjuvant medications play a crucial role in pain management, particularly for neuropathic and chronic pain conditions.*

*These agents, though not primarily analgesics, enhance pain relief and target specific pain mechanisms.*

**Anticonvulsants**
- **Mechanism of Action**: Modulate neuronal excitability and inhibit abnormal electrical discharges in nerves.
- **Common Examples**: Gabapentin, pregabalin, carbamazepine.
- **Indications**: Effective for neuropathic pain conditions such as diabetic neuropathy, postherpetic neuralgia, and trigeminal neuralgia.

- **Adverse Effects**: Include sedation, dizziness, and peripheral edema. Gradual dose titration helps mitigate side effects.

## Antidepressants

- **Mechanism of Action**: Inhibit the reuptake of serotonin and norepinephrine, enhancing descending inhibitory pain pathways.
- **Common Examples**: Tricyclic antidepressants (amitriptyline, nortriptyline) and serotonin-norepinephrine reuptake inhibitors (SNRIs) such as duloxetine and venlafaxine.
- **Indications**: Neuropathic pain, fibromyalgia, chronic headaches, and other chronic pain conditions.
- **Adverse Effects**: Sedation, dry mouth, weight gain (tricyclics), and sexual dysfunction (SNRIs).

## 3.4 Topical Agents

*Topical medications provide localized pain relief with minimal systemic side effects.*

*They are particularly useful for musculoskeletal pain, localized neuropathic pain, and superficial injuries.*

## Common Topical Agents:

- **Topical NSAIDs (e.g., diclofenac gel)**: Provide local anti-inflammatory and analgesic effects for conditions such as osteoarthritis and tendinitis.
- **Capsaicin Cream**: Derived from chili peppers, it depletes substance P from sensory nerves, reducing pain over time. Used for neuropathic pain, postherpetic neuralgia, and osteoarthritis.

- **Lidocaine Patches**: Provide localized analgesia for conditions such as postherpetic neuralgia. Lidocaine reduces sodium channel activity, inhibiting pain signal transmission.

## 3.5 Pharmacokinetics And Considerations For Special Populations

**Pharmacokinetics in Pain Management**: *Understanding the absorption, distribution, metabolism, and excretion (ADME) of pain medications is essential for safe and effective therapy, especially in patients with comorbid conditions.*

## Special Populations:

- **Elderly Patients**: Reduced renal and hepatic function may necessitate dose adjustments and careful monitoring for drug interactions.
- **Pediatric Patients**: Special attention to age-appropriate formulations, dosing, and risk of adverse effects is critical.
- **Renal and Hepatic Impairment**: Dose adjustments or alternative medications may be needed due to altered metabolism and excretion.
- **Pregnant and Breastfeeding Women**: Certain analgesics are contraindicated or must be used with caution to avoid potential teratogenic effects or neonatal complications.

# CHAPTER 4: NON-PHARMACOLOGICAL THERAPIES FOR PAIN MANAGEMENT

## 4.1 Physical Therapy And Rehabilitation

**Physical therapy (PT)** *focuses on restoring physical function and movement through targeted exercises, manual techniques, and other modalities.*

*It plays a vital role in the treatment and rehabilitation of patients with acute, chronic, or post-surgical pain.*

- **Therapeutic Exercise**: Programs tailored to individual needs can strengthen muscles, improve joint mobility, and promote better posture. Examples include stretching, strengthening, and endurance training exercises. Exercise therapy is particularly effective for conditions such as chronic low back pain, osteoarthritis, and fibromyalgia.
- **Manual Therapy**: This includes hands-on techniques such as joint mobilization, manipulation, and soft tissue massage aimed at reducing pain, improving range of motion, and decreasing muscle tension.
- **Modalities**: These are adjunct treatments that can enhance pain relief. Examples include:
  - **Heat and Cold Therapy**: Heat can help relax tense muscles and improve circulation, while cold can reduce inflammation and numb sore tissues.
  - **Electrical Stimulation (e.g., TENS):**

Transcutaneous electrical nerve stimulation (TENS) delivers low-voltage electrical currents to modulate pain signals.
- **Ultrasound Therapy**: Uses high-frequency sound waves to promote tissue healing and reduce inflammation.

**Role of Rehabilitation**: *Rehabilitation focuses on helping patients return to their daily activities, maintain independence, and prevent further injury.*

*Physical therapists often collaborate with other healthcare professionals to create comprehensive treatment plans.*

## 4.2 Occupational Therapy Approaches

**Occupational therapy (OT)** *aims to enable patients to perform daily activities and maintain or regain their independence despite pain.*

*It emphasizes adapting environments and teaching skills to improve function and quality of life.*

- **Activity Modification**: Occupational therapists work with patients to modify tasks or environments to reduce pain. For example, using ergonomic tools, adjusting workstations, and pacing daily activities can reduce physical strain.
- **Energy Conservation Techniques**: Patients with chronic pain are taught methods to balance activity and rest, thereby preventing overexertion and flare-ups of pain.
- **Adaptive Equipment**: Tools such as braces, splints, or assistive devices can alleviate pain and improve function, particularly for patients with arthritis or repetitive strain injuries.

- **Pain Coping Strategies**: Occupational therapists help patients develop skills to manage their pain and overcome barriers to participating in meaningful activities.

## 4.3 Psychological Therapies (Cbt, Mindfulness, Biofeedback)

**Chronic pain** often has a significant psychological component, and addressing this aspect is crucial for effective pain management.

Psychological therapies can alter pain perception, improve coping mechanisms, and reduce the impact of pain on daily life.

- **Cognitive Behavioral Therapy (CBT)**:
    - **Overview**: CBT is a structured, time-limited therapy that focuses on identifying and changing negative thought patterns and behaviors that contribute to the pain experience.
    - **Benefits**: CBT can help patients reframe how they perceive pain, develop healthy coping skills, and reduce feelings of depression or anxiety that often accompany chronic pain.
    - **Components**: Includes cognitive restructuring, relaxation techniques, behavioral activation, and goal setting.
- **Mindfulness-Based Stress Reduction (MBSR)**:
    - **Overview**: Mindfulness involves paying attention to the present moment without judgment. It can reduce pain perception, stress, and negative emotional responses.
    - **Benefits**: Evidence shows that mindfulness

can lower pain intensity and improve quality of life in conditions such as chronic low back pain and fibromyalgia.
- **Biofeedback**:
    - **Overview**: Biofeedback involves using sensors to monitor physiological functions (e.g., heart rate, muscle tension) and providing real-time feedback to the patient.
    - **Benefits**: Patients learn to control and regulate these functions, thereby reducing pain and stress. Biofeedback is often used for tension headaches, migraines, and chronic musculoskeletal pain.

## 4.4 Complementary And Alternative Medicine (Cam)

- **Acupuncture**:
    - **Overview**: A traditional Chinese medicine practice that involves inserting thin needles into specific points on the body to restore balance and promote healing.
    - **Mechanism**: Acupuncture is thought to stimulate the release of endorphins, serotonin, and other neurochemicals that modulate pain.
    - **Evidence and Applications**: Studies have demonstrated benefits for conditions such as chronic pain, migraines, osteoarthritis, and low back pain.
- **Chiropractic Care**:
    - **Overview**: Focuses on diagnosing and treating mechanical disorders of the

musculoskeletal system, especially the spine, through manual adjustment and manipulation.
- ◦ **Benefits**: Chiropractic treatment may relieve back and neck pain, headaches, and joint discomfort through spinal adjustments and mobilization techniques.
- **Massage Therapy**:
  - ◦ **Overview**: Massage involves the manipulation of soft tissues to reduce muscle tension, enhance circulation, and promote relaxation.
  - ◦ **Applications**: Effective for chronic pain conditions such as fibromyalgia, tension headaches, and musculoskeletal injuries.
- **Yoga and Tai Chi**:
  - ◦ **Overview**: These mind-body practices combine physical movement, breath control, and meditation.
  - ◦ **Benefits**: Yoga and tai chi can improve flexibility, strength, balance, and mental well-being while reducing pain in chronic conditions like arthritis and back pain.

**Integration of CAM**: *When considering CAM therapies, it is important to evaluate the evidence base, ensure the approach is safe for the patient, and maintain open communication between all healthcare providers involved in the patient's care.*

# CHAPTER 5: INTERVENTIONAL PAIN MANAGEMENT TECHNIQUES

## 5.1 Nerve Blocks And Injections (E.g., Epidural Steroid Injections)

*Nerve blocks involve the injection of medications such as anesthetics or anti-inflammatory agents near specific nerves or bundles of nerves to interrupt pain signaling pathways.*

- **Epidural Steroid Injections (ESI):**
    - **Overview**: An ESI delivers corticosteroids and sometimes local anesthetics into the epidural space surrounding the spinal cord.
    - **Indications**: Commonly used for radicular pain caused by conditions such as herniated discs, spinal stenosis, and sciatica.
    - **Mechanism of Action**: Corticosteroids reduce inflammation, while anesthetics provide immediate pain relief by numbing the affected area.
    - **Procedure**: Performed under fluoroscopic guidance to ensure accurate placement of the injection.
    - **Risks and Benefits**: Potential complications include infection, bleeding, nerve damage, and transient increases in pain. However, many patients experience significant symptom relief, allowing for improved

function and reduced reliance on medications.
- **Facet Joint Injections**:
  - **Indications**: Used to diagnose and treat pain originating from the facet joints, often related to arthritis or spine degeneration.
  - **Technique**: Involves the injection of anesthetics and corticosteroids into the affected joint.
  - **Benefits**: Can reduce pain and inflammation and help determine if the facet joint is the primary pain source.
- **Peripheral Nerve Blocks**:
  - **Applications**: Used for pain management in specific areas, such as nerve pain following surgery or trauma, or for chronic regional pain syndrome (CRPS).
  - **Mechanism**: Temporarily disrupts nerve function, reducing the transmission of pain signals.

**Clinical Considerations**:

*Nerve blocks can be diagnostic, therapeutic, or both.*

*In many cases, they help identify pain sources and inform subsequent treatment plans.*

## 5.2 Radiofrequency Ablation (Rfa)

**Radiofrequency Ablation (RFA)** *involves using heat generated by radiofrequency energy to target specific nerves, interrupting their ability to transmit pain signals.*

- **Procedure Overview**:
  - **Technique**: A needle is inserted under

imaging guidance (e.g., fluoroscopy or ultrasound) to the target nerve, and radiofrequency energy is applied to generate heat.
- **Applications**: RFA is commonly used for chronic pain conditions such as facet joint pain, sacroiliac joint pain, and peripheral nerve pain.
- **Benefits**: Pain relief from RFA can last from several months to a year or longer, allowing for reduced medication use and improved function.
- **Risks and Side Effects**: Potential risks include local pain, nerve injury, bleeding, and infection. The procedure is minimally invasive and typically performed on an outpatient basis.

**Mechanism of Pain Relief**: *RFA interrupts the nerve's ability to transmit pain signals to the brain by creating a heat lesion, leading to reduced pain perception.*

## 5.3 Spinal Cord Stimulation (Scs)

*Spinal cord stimulation involves the implantation of a device that sends electrical impulses to the spinal cord to modulate pain signals before they reach the brain.*

- **Indications**:
  - **Chronic Pain**: Often used for conditions such as failed back surgery syndrome, complex regional pain syndrome (CRPS), and chronic neuropathic pain.
  - **Refractory Pain**: Considered when conservative treatments have failed or for patients seeking alternatives to long-term

opioid use.
- **Procedure**:
    - **Trial Period**: Patients typically undergo a trial implantation of a temporary stimulator to evaluate its effectiveness before permanent implantation.
    - **Implantation**: If successful, a permanent device consisting of a pulse generator and electrodes is implanted.
- **Mechanism of Action**: Electrical impulses are delivered to the spinal cord, altering pain signal transmission and often replacing it with a tingling sensation known as paresthesia.
- **Benefits**:
    - Provides significant pain relief for many patients.
    - Reduces the need for high doses of pain medications.
    - Improves quality of life and function.
- **Risks**: Complications may include device malfunction, infection, electrode migration, or inadequate pain relief. However, advancements in device technology continue to improve safety and efficacy.

## 5.4 Intrathecal Drug Delivery Systems

*Intrathecal drug delivery systems, also known as pain pumps, involve the placement of a small pump that delivers medication directly into the cerebrospinal fluid surrounding the spinal cord.*

- **Mechanism and Benefits**:
    - **Direct Delivery**: By bypassing systemic circulation, intrathecal drug delivery allows for smaller doses of medication with fewer

systemic side effects.

- **Medications**: Typically used for opioids, local anesthetics, or other agents to manage chronic pain or spasticity.
- **Applications**: Effective for patients with cancer pain, chronic non-cancer pain, or spasticity that has not responded well to oral or systemic therapies.

- **Procedure**:
  - **Implantation**: The device is surgically placed under the skin, and a catheter is inserted into the intrathecal space.
  - **Programming**: The pump is programmed to deliver a precise dose of medication based on patient needs.

- **Considerations**:
  - **Safety**: Intrathecal delivery reduces systemic side effects and improves pain control but requires careful monitoring and follow-up.
  - **Risks**: Potential risks include infection, catheter-related complications, overdose, and device malfunction.

**Integrating Interventional Techniques**: *Interventional procedures, when used in conjunction with other therapies, can provide significant relief for chronic pain sufferers. Proper patient selection, informed consent, and an interdisciplinary approach are critical to optimizing outcomes and minimizing risks.*

# CHAPTER 6: SURGICAL APPROACHES TO PAIN MANAGEMENT

## 6.1 Indications For Pain-Related Surgery

*Pain-related surgeries are typically considered when less invasive treatments have proven ineffective, and the patient's quality of life is significantly impaired by chronic pain.*

*Appropriate patient selection and thorough preoperative evaluations are crucial to achieving favorable outcomes.*

*Indications for pain-related surgery include:*

- **Persistent and Severe Chronic Pain**: Pain that has not responded to pharmacological, physical, or minimally invasive interventions.
- **Structural Abnormalities**: Conditions such as herniated discs, spinal stenosis, or joint degeneration that cause pain due to anatomical changes.
- **Nerve Compression or Damage**: Surgical decompression may be necessary for conditions like nerve root impingement, carpal tunnel syndrome, or peripheral nerve entrapment.
- **Cancer Pain**: Palliative surgical interventions, such as nerve ablation, may be indicated to manage intractable pain from cancer or tumor infiltration.
- **Refractory Neuropathic Pain**: In cases where neurostimulation or other therapies have been ineffective, surgical solutions may offer relief.

**Preoperative Considerations**: *Surgical intervention should be guided by a multidisciplinary team and informed by the patient's overall health, prognosis, and preferences.*

## 6.2 Neurostimulation And Neurosurgical Procedures

*Neurostimulation and neurosurgical interventions directly modulate pain pathways within the nervous system.*

*Key approaches include:*

- **Spinal Cord Stimulation (SCS)**:
    - **Description**: A small device implanted under the skin delivers electrical impulses to the spinal cord, modulating pain signals before they reach the brain.
    - **Indications**: Chronic back and leg pain, complex regional pain syndrome (CRPS), and post-surgical neuropathic pain.
    - **Procedure**: Typically involves a trial period with a temporary stimulator to assess efficacy before permanent implantation.
    - **Benefits and Risks**: SCS often reduces pain and the need for medication, but potential complications include device migration, infection, and hardware malfunctions.
- **Deep Brain Stimulation (DBS)**:
    - **Mechanism**: Electrodes are placed in specific areas of the brain to modulate neural activity and alleviate pain.
    - **Applications**: Rarely used but can be effective

for intractable pain syndromes and certain types of neuropathic pain.
- **Motor Cortex Stimulation:**
  - **Overview**: Electrical stimulation applied to the motor cortex has shown promise for neuropathic pain, including post-stroke or trigeminal neuropathies.
- **Dorsal Root Ganglion (DRG) Stimulation:**
  - **Description**: Targets sensory nerves near the spinal cord to precisely modulate pain signals.
  - **Benefits**: Effective for focal neuropathic pain, including CRPS.
- **Neurosurgical Ablation:**
  - **Overview**: Targeted destruction of pain-transmitting nerves or brain pathways (e.g., cordotomy, cingulotomy).
  - **Indications**: Reserved for patients with severe, intractable pain and limited life expectancy.

## 6.3 Orthopedic And Spine Surgeries For Pain

*Surgical interventions on the musculoskeletal system may be indicated when structural abnormalities lead to chronic pain:*

- **Spinal Surgeries:**
  - **Discectomy/Microdiscectomy**: Removal of herniated disc material that is pressing on a nerve root.
  - **Laminectomy/Decompression Surgery**: Removal of bone and tissue to relieve pressure on the spinal cord or nerves.
  - **Spinal Fusion**: Joining two or more vertebrae

to stabilize the spine and alleviate pain from conditions such as degenerative disc disease or spondylolisthesis.
- **Artificial Disc Replacement**: An alternative to fusion, where a damaged disc is replaced with an artificial one to maintain motion and reduce pain.
- **Orthopedic Surgeries**:
  - **Joint Replacement (Arthroplasty)**: Replacing damaged joints (e.g., hip, knee) with prosthetic implants for pain relief in severe arthritis.
  - **Arthroscopic Procedures**: Minimally invasive procedures to treat joint pain due to cartilage tears, inflammation, or loose fragments.
  - **Osteotomy**: Cutting and realigning bones to relieve pain and improve function in conditions like knee arthritis.

**Considerations**: *Careful assessment of patient expectations, comorbidities, and rehabilitation needs is essential for successful outcomes.*

## 6.4 Postoperative Pain Management Strategies

*Strategies include:*

- **Multimodal Analgesia**: Combining different classes of medications (e.g., NSAIDs, opioids, local anesthetics) to target various pain pathways, minimizing the need for

high-dose opioids.
- **Regional Anesthesia and Nerve Blocks**:
    - **Epidural Analgesia**: Continuous infusion of local anesthetic and/or opioids via an epidural catheter.
    - **Peripheral Nerve Blocks**: Provide targeted pain relief and reduce the need for systemic analgesics.
- **Patient-Controlled Analgesia (PCA)**:
    - **Description**: Allows patients to self-administer small doses of pain medication, offering a sense of control and timely pain relief.
- **Non-Pharmacological Techniques**:
    - **Physical Therapy**: Encourages mobility, reduces stiffness, and prevents complications such as deep vein thrombosis.
    - **Psychological Support**: Cognitive-behavioral strategies, mindfulness, and relaxation techniques can enhance recovery and reduce postoperative anxiety.

# CHAPTER 7: CHRONIC PAIN MANAGEMENT STRATEGIES

*Chronic pain, persisting for months or even years, significantly impacts patients' quality of life, mental health, and daily functioning.*

## 7.1 Managing Chronic Non-Cancer Pain

*Chronic non-cancer pain (CNCP) includes conditions like chronic low back pain, osteoarthritis, chronic headache disorders, and musculoskeletal pain syndromes.*

*Key management strategies involve:*

- **Multidisciplinary Care**:
    - Involvement of various healthcare professionals, including primary care providers, pain specialists, physical therapists, psychologists, and occupational therapists.
    - Development of individualized care plans tailored to patients' needs and goals.
- **Pharmacological Management**:
    - **Non-Opioid Analgesics**: NSAIDs, acetaminophen, and topical analgesics are first-line agents.
    - **Opioids**: Used cautiously, with strict monitoring to balance benefits and risks, particularly the risk of dependency and opioid-induced hyperalgesia.
    - **Adjuvants**: Antidepressants (e.g., tricyclics,

SNRIs) and anticonvulsants (e.g., gabapentin, pregabalin) for neuropathic and other complex pain syndromes.
- **Behavioral and Psychological Interventions**:
    - **Cognitive Behavioral Therapy (CBT)**: Focuses on changing maladaptive thoughts and behaviors associated with chronic pain.
    - **Mindfulness-Based Stress Reduction (MBSR)**: Promotes awareness of pain without emotional attachment, reducing stress and improving coping mechanisms.
- **Non-Pharmacological Therapies**:
    - **Exercise Therapy**: Individualized programs to improve strength, flexibility, and endurance.
    - **Physical Therapy**: Manual therapies, heat/cold applications, and transcutaneous electrical nerve stimulation (TENS).
    - **Complementary Therapies**: Acupuncture, massage, and other alternative approaches may offer relief for some patients.

## 7.2 Pain Management In Cancer Patients

*Key principles include:*

- **Assessment**:
    - Comprehensive assessment of pain, including etiology (nociceptive, neuropathic, mixed), severity, and impact on daily living.
    - Regular re-evaluation to adapt strategies as the patient's condition changes.
- **Pharmacological Therapies**:
    - **WHO Analgesic Ladder**: A stepwise approach

starting with non-opioid analgesics and progressing to opioids for moderate to severe pain, with adjuvants as needed.
- **Opioids**: Mainstay for moderate to severe cancer pain, including morphine, oxycodone, and fentanyl. Close monitoring for side effects and tolerance is essential.
- **Adjuvant Therapies**: Antidepressants, anticonvulsants, corticosteroids, bisphosphonates, and radiopharmaceuticals for specific pain types.
- Interventional Approaches:
  - **Nerve Blocks**: Targeted nerve blocks to alleviate localized pain.
  - **Intrathecal Pumps**: Deliver medications directly to the cerebrospinal fluid for severe, refractory pain.
  - **Palliative Radiotherapy**: For pain relief from bone metastases or tumors causing pressure.
- Psychological Support:
  - Addressing psychological distress, anxiety, and depression that often accompany cancer-related pain.
  - Use of support groups, counseling, and relaxation techniques.

## 7.3 Strategies For Neuropathic Pain

*Key strategies for management include:*

- **Pharmacological Therapies**:
  - **First-Line Agents**: Anticonvulsants such as gabapentin and pregabalin; antidepressants

like amitriptyline, duloxetine, or venlafaxine.
- **Topical Agents**: Lidocaine patches and capsaicin cream can be effective for localized neuropathic pain.
- **Second-Line Options**: Opioids (cautiously), tramadol, or combination therapies for refractory cases.
- **Non-Pharmacological Approaches**:
    - **Physical Therapy**: Focuses on restoring function, improving gait and posture, and reducing deconditioning.
    - **Psychological Therapies**: Address the emotional impact of chronic neuropathic pain.
- **Interventional Therapies**:
    - **Nerve Blocks**: Diagnostic or therapeutic injections to target specific nerve pain.
    - **Spinal Cord Stimulation**: Provides effective pain relief in refractory cases of neuropathic pain.

## 7.4 Central Sensitization And Fibromyalgia

*Central sensitization is characterized by an amplification of pain signals in the central nervous system, often resulting in widespread pain, hyperalgesia, and fatigue.*

*Fibromyalgia is a prominent example of a central sensitization disorder.*

- **Diagnosis**:
    - Diagnostic criteria focus on widespread musculoskeletal pain lasting for more than three months, with associated symptoms like fatigue, sleep disturbances, and cognitive

difficulties.
- **Management Approaches**:
  - **Pharmacological Therapies**: Tricyclic antidepressants (e.g., amitriptyline), SNRIs (e.g., duloxetine), and anticonvulsants (e.g., pregabalin) are commonly used.
  - **Non-Pharmacological Therapies**:
    - **Exercise Programs**: Aerobic exercise, strengthening, and stretching have proven benefits in reducing pain and improving function.
    - **CBT and Stress Management**: Help patients manage the psychological impact of chronic pain.
    - **Complementary Approaches**: Acupuncture, tai chi, and mindfulness meditation may provide symptom relief.
- **Patient Education**:
  - Empowering patients with knowledge about their condition, realistic expectations, and coping strategies is essential for effective management.

# CHAPTER 8: PEDIATRIC PAIN MANAGEMENT

## 8.1 Assessment And Unique Considerations In Children

**Accurate Pain Assessment** *is crucial in pediatric patients to ensure appropriate and effective management. Unlike adults, children may have difficulty expressing their pain clearly, making assessment challenging.*

*Key approaches include:*

- **Developmentally Appropriate Pain Assessment Tools**:
    - **Neonates and Infants**: Use observational tools such as the **Neonatal Infant Pain Scale (NIPS)**, which assesses facial expression, crying, breathing patterns, arm and leg movements, and arousal state.
    - **Toddlers and Preschoolers**: The **FLACC Scale (Face, Legs, Activity, Cry, Consolability)** can be helpful for young children unable to communicate their pain verbally.
    - **School-Age Children**: **Visual Analog Scales (VAS)** or the **Faces Pain Scale–Revised (FPS-R)** allow children to self-report pain by pointing to a series of faces ranging from happy (no pain) to distressed (severe pain).
    - **Adolescents**: Utilize numeric rating scales (0–10) similar to adults, provided they

understand the concept.
- **Psychosocial and Cultural Influences on Pain**:
    - **Parental and Caregiver Presence**: The influence of caregivers' attitudes toward pain, along with cultural norms around pain expression, can impact how children respond to and report pain.
    - **Anxiety and Fear**: Addressing a child's fear of pain, particularly for procedures, is essential. Pre-procedural preparation, distraction techniques, and providing reassurance are vital steps.
- **Developmental and Physiological Considerations**:
    - **Pharmacokinetic Differences**: Drug metabolism and clearance rates differ in children, necessitating careful dosing based on age, weight, and development stage.
    - **Pain Memory**: Experiences of poorly managed acute pain may contribute to chronic pain syndromes in children, making early and effective intervention essential.

## 8.2 Pharmacological Approaches To Pediatric Pain Management

**Pharmacological interventions** should be chosen and dosed with care, given children's unique physiological and developmental needs.

*Key categories include:*
- **Non-Opioid Analgesics**:
    - **Acetaminophen** and **NSAIDs (e.g., ibuprofen)** are often first-line agents for mild to moderate pain. Weight-based dosing is

essential to avoid toxicity.
- **Caution with Aspirin**: Aspirin should generally be avoided in children due to the risk of Reye's syndrome.

- **Opioid Analgesics**:
  - **Indications and Dosing**: Reserved for moderate to severe pain, opioids like morphine and hydromorphone must be carefully dosed and monitored.
  - **Risk Management**: Close monitoring for respiratory depression, sedation, and other adverse effects is necessary, especially in opioid-naïve children.
  - **Opioid-Sparing Approaches**: Combining opioids with non-opioids or adjuvants can reduce required doses and minimize side effects.

- **Adjuvant Medications**:
  - **Anticonvulsants (e.g., gabapentin)** for neuropathic pain.
  - **Antidepressants** may be considered in chronic pain syndromes, particularly when associated with anxiety or depression.

## 8.3 Non-Pharmacological Approaches

- **Physical Therapies**:
  - **Positioning and Splinting**: Proper positioning and immobilization can reduce musculoskeletal pain.
  - **Exercise and Movement Therapy**: Tailored physical therapy programs help improve function and reduce chronic pain in children

with musculoskeletal disorders.
- **Psychological Therapies**:
    - **Cognitive Behavioral Therapy (CBT)**: CBT can help children identify and manage negative thoughts about pain, develop coping strategies, and improve overall functioning.
    - **Distraction Techniques**: Guided imagery, storytelling, virtual reality games, and breathing exercises can be effective during painful procedures.
    - **Biofeedback**: Used to teach children to control physiological processes, such as heart rate and muscle tension, which may influence pain perception.
- **Complementary and Alternative Medicine (CAM)**:
    - **Acupuncture**: Evidence supports acupuncture for some types of chronic pain in children.
    - **Massage Therapy**: Helps reduce tension, anxiety, and pain perception.
    - **Music Therapy and Art Therapy**: Provide distraction and a means for emotional expression.
- **Family Involvement**:
    - **Parental Support**: Educating parents and involving them in the pain management plan can reduce children's anxiety and improve adherence to therapies.
    - **Caregiver Training**: Parents can be taught techniques to provide comfort and distraction during painful procedures at home.

# CHAPTER 9: GERIATRIC PAIN MANAGEMENT

## 9.1 Challenges In The Elderly Population

*Pain management in geriatric patients must account for a variety of complexities:*

- **Age-Related Physiological Changes**:
    - **Altered Pain Perception**: The elderly may exhibit differences in pain thresholds and tolerance, leading to underreporting of pain.
    - **Decreased Renal and Hepatic Function**: Age-related decline in organ function affects drug metabolism and excretion, increasing the risk of toxicity and adverse effects.
    - **Cognitive Impairment**: Conditions such as dementia can make pain assessment difficult, as patients may be unable to articulate their discomfort. Behavioral indicators like restlessness, grimacing, or withdrawal may provide clues.
- **Comorbidities**:
    - Older adults often have multiple chronic conditions (e.g., cardiovascular disease, diabetes, osteoarthritis), which can complicate pain management strategies and limit treatment options.
- **Social and Economic Factors**:
    - **Social Isolation**: Many elderly patients live

alone or are socially isolated, potentially exacerbating feelings of helplessness and negatively impacting pain perception.
- **Financial Barriers**: Fixed incomes may limit access to certain therapies, medications, or healthcare services.

## 9.2 Polypharmacy And Drug Interactions

**Polypharmacy**—*the use of multiple medications—is common in elderly patients, increasing the risk of drug interactions and side effects that complicate pain management.*

*Key considerations include:*

- **Medication Reviews**:
  - **Regular Assessment**: A thorough medication history and periodic reviews can help minimize inappropriate prescriptions, identify drug interactions, and optimize therapy.
  - **Beers Criteria**: Utilize evidence-based guidelines (e.g., Beers Criteria) to identify potentially inappropriate medications in older adults and reduce the risk of adverse outcomes.
- **Risk of Adverse Drug Reactions (ADRs)**:
  - **Non-Opioid Analgesics**: NSAIDs may cause gastrointestinal bleeding, kidney dysfunction, or cardiovascular issues, especially in prolonged use. Acetaminophen is generally safer but must be monitored to prevent liver toxicity.
  - **Opioid Therapy**: While opioids can be effective for moderate-to-severe pain, older

adults are more susceptible to side effects such as sedation, constipation, falls, and respiratory depression. Careful titration and monitoring are essential.
- **CYP Enzyme Interactions**: Many medications metabolized by cytochrome P450 enzymes can interact with pain medications, leading to increased or decreased efficacy.
- **Balancing Pain Relief and Safety**:
    - **Dose Adjustments**: Start with low doses and titrate slowly to achieve the desired effect while minimizing risks.
    - **Use of Adjuvant Medications**: Anticonvulsants and antidepressants may be beneficial for neuropathic pain but should be chosen with caution due to potential side effects (e.g., sedation, dizziness).

## 9.3 Psychological And Functional Considerations

*Addressing psychological and functional factors is essential in geriatric pain management:*

- **Psychological Considerations**:
    - **Depression and Anxiety**: Chronic pain often coexists with depression and anxiety, complicating treatment. Effective management requires a comprehensive approach that may involve psychotherapy, antidepressants, and/or supportive counseling.
    - **Fear of Addiction**: Older adults may have fears or misconceptions about pain medications, particularly opioids, which may lead to underutilization. Providing education

and reassurance about pain management options is crucial.
- **Functional Considerations:**
  - **Mobility and Balance:** Pain, especially in conditions such as osteoarthritis or chronic back pain, can lead to reduced mobility, falls, and subsequent injury. Functional assessments and balance training should be part of the care plan.
  - **Rehabilitation Strategies:**
    - **Physical Therapy:** Tailored exercise programs help improve strength, flexibility, and overall function while reducing pain.
    - **Assistive Devices:** Walkers, canes, and other assistive devices can enhance mobility and reduce the risk of falls.
  - **Occupational Therapy:** Focuses on adapting activities of daily living (ADLs) and home environments to improve independence and quality of life.
- **Non-Pharmacological Approaches:**
  - **Cognitive Behavioral Therapy (CBT):** CBT can help elderly patients modify their perception of pain, develop coping strategies, and reduce pain-related distress.
  - **Complementary Therapies:** Techniques such as tai chi, yoga, acupuncture, and mindfulness meditation may be effective for certain types of chronic pain.

# CHAPTER 10: PAIN MANAGEMENT IN SPECIAL POPULATIONS

## 10.1 Pain In Patients With Substance Use Disorders

*Managing pain in individuals with **substance use disorders (SUD)** presents a delicate challenge, as these patients may have complex histories of addiction and may be at increased risk of opioid misuse, dependence, or overdose.*

- **Pain Assessment**:
    - **Comprehensive History**: A thorough pain assessment and careful history-taking are essential. This includes understanding the patient's substance use history, including any past or current opioid use, and the type and severity of their pain.
    - **Objective and Subjective Pain Evaluation**: Relying on a combination of subjective reporting and objective measures (e.g., physical examination, imaging) can help differentiate between pain that requires treatment and that which may be exacerbated by addiction behaviors.
- **Pharmacological Management**:
    - **Opioid Alternatives**: For patients with opioid use disorder (OUD), the use of non-opioid analgesics, including **NSAIDs, acetaminophen, anticonvulsants** (e.g., gabapentin), and **antidepressants** (e.g., amitriptyline) can help manage pain without

the risk of opioid misuse.
- **Opioid Agonist Therapy**: In certain cases, **methadone** or **buprenorphine** may be used as part of opioid agonist therapy for managing both pain and addiction, ensuring safe and controlled opioid use.
- **Multimodal Approach**: Combining pharmacological treatments with non-pharmacological approaches, such as cognitive-behavioral therapy (CBT), physical therapy, and alternative medicine (e.g., acupuncture), can reduce the need for opioid analgesics and improve pain control.

- **Psychosocial Considerations**:
  - **Counseling and Support**: Behavioral therapies, including **CBT** and **contingency management**, can be helpful in addressing the psychological aspects of substance use and pain.
  - **Close Monitoring**: Patients with substance use disorders should be closely monitored for signs of misuse, diversion, and overdose when opioids are prescribed, if necessary.

## 10.2 Pain Management In Pregnancy

*Pain management during pregnancy requires careful consideration of both the **maternal** and **fetal** well-being, as certain pain management options can pose risks to the developing fetus.*

*Thus, pharmacological and non-pharmacological approaches must be selected with caution.*

- **Pharmacological Considerations**:

- **Acetaminophen**: Generally considered safe for short-term use during pregnancy for mild to moderate pain.
- **Non-Steroidal Anti-Inflammatory Drugs (NSAIDs)**: NSAIDs should be used with caution, particularly in the third trimester, due to potential risks of premature closure of the ductus arteriosus, oligohydramnios, and renal impairment in the fetus.
- **Opioids**: The use of opioids (e.g., morphine, oxycodone) during pregnancy should be limited to cases of severe pain that cannot be managed with other options. Long-term opioid use can increase the risk of neonatal abstinence syndrome (NAS) and other neonatal complications.
- **Local Anesthetics**: Epidural and spinal anesthesia are common choices for pain relief during labor and delivery, with minimal fetal risk. However, their use must be tailored to the individual's medical and obstetric history.

- **Non-Pharmacological Approaches**:
  - **Physical Therapies**: Techniques such as prenatal massage, physical therapy, and safe exercise can help relieve musculoskeletal pain common during pregnancy (e.g., back pain, pelvic pain).
  - **Cognitive and Behavioral Techniques**: Relaxation exercises, guided imagery, breathing techniques, and **hypnotherapy** are effective in managing labor pain and reducing anxiety.
- **Psychosocial and Emotional Support**:
  - **Education and Preparation**: Providing

pregnant patients with information about pain management options during labor and delivery can help reduce anxiety and allow for better decision-making.
- **Support Systems**: Encouraging the presence of a partner or doula during labor can provide emotional and physical support, which may improve pain tolerance.

## 10.3 Pain In Patients With Mental Health Disorders

*Patients with **mental health disorders**, such as depression, anxiety, and chronic pain syndromes, often have a complicated experience of pain that can be influenced by psychological factors, leading to an exacerbation of both pain and mental health symptoms.*

- **Pain Assessment**:
    - **Comprehensive Pain History**: Patients with mental health disorders may have different pain thresholds and responses to treatment. A careful assessment should consider both physical and emotional factors that may be influencing pain perception.
    - **Multidimensional Pain Screening**: Using tools like the **Brief Pain Inventory (BPI)** or the **McGill Pain Questionnaire** can help assess the sensory, emotional, and cognitive aspects of pain, which is important in patients with psychiatric conditions.
- **Psychiatric Considerations**:
    - **Depression and Pain**: Depression is commonly associated with chronic pain conditions. Antidepressants (e.g., **SSRIs**, **SNRIs**) can not only help treat depression but may also alleviate some types of pain,

particularly **neuropathic pain**.
- **Anxiety and Pain**: Anxiety disorders can exacerbate pain perception and reduce the effectiveness of pain management strategies. **Benzodiazepines** should be used with caution due to their addictive potential and should generally be reserved for short-term use in acute pain situations.
- **Somatization and Pain**: Some patients with psychiatric conditions may have **somatization** (the expression of psychological distress through physical symptoms), which can make pain management more difficult. These patients require careful evaluation to differentiate between physical and psychological causes of pain.

- **Pharmacological Management**:
  - **Antidepressants and Anticonvulsants**: **Tricyclic antidepressants** (e.g., amitriptyline) and anticonvulsants (e.g., gabapentin, pregabalin) are often used to manage neuropathic pain and can be effective in patients with comorbid psychiatric disorders.
  - **Opioid Use in Mental Health Patients**: Caution is required when prescribing opioids, especially in patients with a history of substance use disorder or those at risk of developing dependence.
- **Psychological Therapies**:
  - **Cognitive Behavioral Therapy (CBT)**: CBT has been shown to be effective in managing both chronic pain and the psychological factors

that contribute to or exacerbate pain.

- **Mindfulness and Relaxation**: Techniques such as **mindfulness meditation**, **relaxation training**, and **biofeedback** can reduce the emotional and physiological aspects of pain, leading to better outcomes in patients with co-occurring pain and mental health disorders.

# CHAPTER 11: REGULATORY AND ETHICAL CONSIDERATIONS

## 11.1 Prescription Drug Monitoring Programs (Pdmps)

*Prescription Drug Monitoring Programs (PDMPs) are state-run electronic databases that track the prescribing and dispensing of controlled substances.*

*PDMPs aim to reduce the misuse of prescription drugs and ensure that medications are prescribed appropriately.*

- **Purpose and Function**:
    - PDMPs provide healthcare providers with a real-time history of patients' prescriptions for controlled substances, including opioids, benzodiazepines, and other potentially addictive medications. This allows providers to **identify potential drug misuse** or **doctor shopping** (patients visiting multiple doctors to obtain prescriptions).
    - PDMPs can help **prevent opioid abuse**, **identify patients at risk**, and ensure **safe prescribing practices**.
- **Legal Requirements**:
    - Healthcare providers are typically required by law to check the PDMP database before prescribing controlled substances, particularly opioids, to ensure the patient is

not receiving overlapping prescriptions from multiple sources.
- In some states, PDMPs are mandatory for all opioid prescriptions, while others may require checks in specific circumstances, such as prescribing a high-dose opioid or for long-term use.
- **Benefits of PDMPs**:
  - **Enhanced patient safety**: By reviewing a patient's medication history, clinicians can make more informed decisions about prescribing controlled substances.
  - **Early identification of misuse**: PDMPs can alert providers to patients who may be at risk of drug misuse, allowing for timely intervention.
  - **Reduction of prescription fraud**: These programs help identify fraudulent prescriptions and prevent illicit activities, such as the diversion of medications.
- **Challenges and Limitations**:
  - **Interstate variations**: While PDMPs are widely implemented, the systems and regulations may vary from state to state, creating potential gaps in coverage and difficulties for providers working across multiple states.
  - **Data accuracy**: The accuracy and timeliness of data entry into PDMPs can sometimes be a concern, leading to possible delays or discrepancies in patient records.

# 11.2 Opioid Stewardship And Managing Risk Of

## Misuse

*The management of pain with opioids has become a critical area of focus due to the opioid crisis.*

*Effective **opioid stewardship** involves careful prescribing, monitoring, and patient education to ensure opioids are used safely and appropriately.*

- **Principles of Opioid Stewardship**:
    - **Patient-Centered Care**: Opioid stewardship requires providers to consider each patient's individual circumstances, balancing the need for pain relief with the risks of opioid misuse, addiction, and overdose.
    - **Multimodal Pain Management**: Where possible, opioids should be used as part of a multimodal approach to pain management, incorporating non-opioid medications, physical therapy, and non-pharmacological strategies.
    - **Patient Education**: It is essential to educate patients on the **risks** of opioid use, the **correct usage** of medications, and the importance of **adhering to prescribed doses** and **not sharing medications** with others.
- **Risk Assessment and Monitoring**:
    - **Risk stratification**: Providers should assess each patient's risk for opioid misuse using tools like the **Opioid Risk Tool (ORT)** or **Current Opioid Misuse Measure (COMM)**. These tools help identify individuals who may be at higher risk of misuse and warrant closer monitoring.
    - **Regular follow-ups**: For patients on chronic

opioid therapy, regular follow-ups, urine drug screening, and PDMP checks should be performed to monitor adherence and detect any potential misuse.

- **Safe Prescribing Guidelines**:
    - **Start low, go slow**: When prescribing opioids, clinicians should begin with the lowest effective dose and consider short-term use for acute pain. **Long-term opioid therapy** should be avoided unless absolutely necessary, and the patient should be reassessed regularly.
    - **Use of immediate-release opioids**: Immediate-release formulations are preferred over extended-release or long-acting opioids to reduce the risk of misuse and overdose.
    - **Co-prescribing naloxone**: In high-risk patients, especially those on long-term opioid therapy or with a history of substance use disorder, co-prescribing **naloxone** (an opioid antagonist) can help reverse the effects of opioid overdose in case of an emergency.
- **Addressing Opioid Addiction**:
    - **Medication-Assisted Treatment (MAT)**: For patients with opioid use disorder, MAT with **methadone**, **buprenorphine**, or **naltrexone** can be an essential component of treatment. MAT can help manage cravings and withdrawal symptoms while supporting long-term recovery.
    - **Referral to addiction specialists**: Patients showing signs of opioid misuse or addiction should be referred to **addiction treatment centers** for specialized care, including

counseling and rehabilitation programs.

## 11.3 Ethical Issues In Pain Management

*Ethical challenges often arise in pain management, particularly when the risks and benefits of treatments conflict or when there is uncertainty about the best course of action.*

*Providers must navigate these ethical dilemmas with care to ensure that patients' rights and well-being are respected while balancing the need for pain relief with the risk of harm.*

- **Balancing Pain Relief with the Risk of Addiction**:
    - One of the primary ethical concerns in pain management is prescribing opioids to patients who may be at risk of **addiction** or **misuse**. Providers must balance the obligation to **relieve suffering** with the responsibility to **prevent harm**, particularly given the opioid epidemic.
    - **Ethical principles** like **beneficence** (doing good) and **non-maleficence** (do no harm) guide this delicate balance. Providers should carefully assess the patient's history, monitor closely, and consider alternative pain management strategies.
- **Autonomy and Informed Consent**:
    - Pain management decisions should involve the patient as a central part of the process. Respect for **autonomy** means giving patients the right to make informed decisions about their treatment options.
    - **Informed consent** involves explaining the risks and benefits of different pain management options, including the potential for opioid dependence, so patients can make

choices based on their personal values and understanding.

- **Palliative Care and End-of-Life Pain**:
  - Ethical issues often arise in the context of **end-of-life care** when managing pain for terminally ill patients. In these cases, **palliative care** providers may face dilemmas regarding the **appropriate use of opioids** to alleviate suffering while ensuring that the goal of care remains comfort rather than prolonging life.
  - The **doctrine of double effect** is often referenced here: it states that providing high doses of pain relief, knowing that it may shorten life, is ethically permissible when the primary intention is to alleviate pain.
- **Cultural and Societal Considerations**:
  - Ethical dilemmas may also arise due to cultural differences in understanding pain and its treatment. For example, some patients may have cultural or religious beliefs that influence their decision to use certain medications or treatments.
  - **Cultural competence** in healthcare providers is essential to ensure that pain management respects the patient's values while providing the most effective treatment options.
- **End-of-Life and Physician-Assisted Death**:
  - In certain jurisdictions, physician-assisted death or euthanasia may raise ethical concerns in patients experiencing unmanageable pain. Healthcare providers must understand the laws governing these issues in their specific location and engage in

compassionate discussions with patients and their families.

# CHAPTER 12: EMERGING TRENDS AND FUTURE DIRECTIONS IN PAIN MANAGEMENT

## 12.1 New Pharmacological Agents And Therapies

- **New Classes of Analgesics**:
    - **TRPV1 (Transient Receptor Potential Vanilloid 1) Antagonists**: TRPV1 receptors are involved in the sensation of heat and pain. Researchers are exploring drugs that block TRPV1 to reduce pain without affecting the central nervous system. These may be particularly useful for managing conditions like **neuropathic pain**, **osteoarthritis**, and **muscle pain**.
    - **Cannabinoid-based Therapies**: While cannabis-based products have been used for pain management for centuries, there is renewed interest in developing **pharmaceutical-grade cannabinoids**. These drugs aim to target the **endocannabinoid system** more effectively to relieve pain in conditions like **chronic pain**, **multiple sclerosis**, and **cancer pain**.
    - **NMDA Receptor Antagonists**: NMDA (N-methyl-D-aspartate) receptors play a crucial role in **central sensitization**, a key mechanism in chronic pain. New agents that target NMDA receptors are being developed to

manage **neuropathic pain** and **fibromyalgia** by preventing pain amplification in the central nervous system.

- **Non-Opioid Analgesics**:
  - **Atypical Analgesics**: Medications such as **nalbuphine**, a kappa-opioid agonist, are being investigated for their ability to relieve pain while having a lower potential for abuse and addiction compared to traditional opioids.
  - **Gene Therapy**: The potential use of gene therapy to **modulate pain pathways** is a growing area of research. By introducing specific genes into the nervous system, it may be possible to **reduce pain sensitivity** or **promote the regeneration of nerve tissue**, offering a novel approach for conditions like **chronic pain** and **neuropathies**.
- **Biologic Therapies**:
  - **Monoclonal Antibodies**: These targeted biologics are being developed to address specific pathways involved in pain, particularly in inflammatory pain conditions like **rheumatoid arthritis** and **complex regional pain syndrome (CRPS)**. Agents targeting **interleukins** and **tumor necrosis factor (TNF)** are already in use for inflammatory diseases and may soon be adapted for pain management.
  - **Stem Cell Therapy**: Stem cells hold the potential to regenerate damaged tissues and alter pain signaling pathways. Early studies are examining the use of **mesenchymal stem cells** (MSCs) to repair nerve damage or promote healing in areas like the **spine** and

joints.

## 12.2 Advances In Neurotechnology And Ai For Pain Assessment

*The use of **neurotechnology** and **artificial intelligence (AI)** is reshaping pain management by providing more precise ways to assess, monitor, and treat pain.*

- **Neurostimulation Devices**:
    - **Transcranial Magnetic Stimulation (TMS)**: This non-invasive technique uses magnetic fields to stimulate specific brain areas involved in pain processing. TMS has shown promise in treating **chronic pain** and **depression** simultaneously and is being explored for use in conditions like **fibromyalgia** and **chronic low back pain**.
    - **Transcutaneous Electrical Nerve Stimulation (TENS)**: TENS devices are already widely used for pain relief. New advancements in TENS, such as **wearable devices** with **adaptive stimulation algorithms**, are enhancing their effectiveness by tailoring the stimulation to the patient's unique pain experience.
- **Implantable Neurostimulators**: These devices deliver electrical impulses to the **spinal cord**, **peripheral nerves**, or **brain** to modulate pain pathways. **Spinal cord stimulation (SCS)** and **deep brain stimulation (DBS)** are becoming more sophisticated, with new models offering more precise control and the ability to target specific areas of the nervous system.
- **AI in Pain Assessment**:

- **Machine Learning Models**: AI algorithms are being developed to analyze vast amounts of patient data (e.g., from wearables, imaging, and electronic health records) to predict pain patterns and **personalize treatment**. These tools can assist healthcare providers in identifying the most effective treatments and detecting early signs of pain flare-ups.
- **Neuroimaging**: Advanced neuroimaging techniques, such as **functional MRI** and **PET scans**, are now being used to study the brain's response to pain. AI can enhance the interpretation of these images, helping to identify biomarkers for **chronic pain** and **neuropathic pain**, which can guide more targeted therapies.

## 12.3 Personalized And Precision Pain Medicine

*The concept of **personalized pain medicine** revolves around tailoring pain management strategies based on a patient's genetic, environmental, and psychosocial factors.*

*As research into the genetic and molecular underpinnings of pain continues to grow, the future of pain management will likely involve highly individualized treatments.*

- **Genetic and Molecular Insights**:
    - **Pain Gene Variability**: Genetic factors play a significant role in how individuals experience pain. Variations in genes related to pain receptors (e.g., **OPRM1** for opioid receptors), neurotransmitters, and ion channels can influence both pain sensitivity and response to treatment. **Pharmacogenetic testing** could

soon be a routine part of pain management, helping doctors prescribe the most effective medications for each patient based on their genetic profile.

- **Biomarkers for Pain**: The identification of biomarkers—molecular signatures that indicate the presence or intensity of pain—could allow clinicians to diagnose and treat pain more precisely. These biomarkers could come from **blood tests**, **urine samples**, or even **genetic testing**.

- **Tailoring Treatment Plans**:
  - **Integrated Treatment**: Personalized pain management involves not just pharmacological interventions but also psychological therapies, physical therapy, and lifestyle adjustments. By understanding the genetic and environmental factors that influence pain perception, clinicians can create **customized treatment plans** that combine the most effective modalities for each patient.
  - **Precision Medicine Platforms**: Companies are working on developing **digital platforms** that aggregate genetic data, health histories, and other personal factors to recommend tailored pain management strategies. These platforms could guide treatment options for chronic pain, ensuring patients receive the most appropriate therapies based on their unique characteristics.

- **Real-time Adaptive Pain Management**:
  - As wearable devices become more advanced, they can continuously monitor pain levels,

physiological responses, and environmental factors, providing real-time data that can be used to adjust treatment plans dynamically. This level of personalization could improve outcomes by allowing for **continuous adjustments** to pain management in response to changing conditions.

# CHAPTER 13: 20 CASE STUDIES AND CLINICAL SCENARIOS

## Case Study 1: Acute Postoperative Pain Management

**Patient**: A 45-year-old woman undergoing total knee replacement.

**Clinical Scenario**: The patient is admitted to the post-anesthesia care unit (PACU) following a total knee replacement.

She reports moderate to severe pain at the surgical site, with a pain score of 8/10 on the visual analogue scale (VAS).

She has a history of mild opioid use for chronic back pain but has no known drug allergies.

**Assessment and Management**:
- **Immediate pain relief**: Initial pain management involves the use of **patient-controlled analgesia (PCA)** with morphine.
- **Multimodal analgesia**: In addition to opioids, a **nerve block** (femoral nerve block) is placed preoperatively to reduce reliance on opioids post-surgery.
- **Postoperative follow-up**: The patient is reassessed every 2 hours, and her opioid use is minimized by using **NSAIDs** (ibuprofen) and **acetaminophen** in combination.

**Outcome**: The patient achieves satisfactory pain relief with reduced opioid consumption and minimal side effects. She is discharged with a tailored analgesic regimen and instructions for physical therapy to facilitate early mobilization.

**Discussion**: The key to effective postoperative pain management in this case lies in the **multimodal approach** that minimizes opioid use while addressing both nociceptive and inflammatory pain components.

## Case Study 2: Chronic Back Pain Management

**Patient**: A 60-year-old male with chronic low back pain (CLBP).

**Clinical Scenario**: The patient presents with a 5-year history of persistent lower back pain.

Despite trying physical therapy, NSAIDs, and occasional epidural steroid injections, his pain has worsened, and he now experiences functional limitations.

**Assessment and Management**:

- **Comprehensive evaluation**: A thorough assessment, including MRI imaging, reveals evidence of **degenerative disc disease** and **facet joint osteoarthritis**.
- **Multidisciplinary management**: The pain management team includes an orthopedic surgeon, a physical therapist, and a pain specialist. A **multimodal pain management plan** is initiated, involving physical therapy, psychological support (CBT for coping with chronic pain), and a **spinal cord stimulator trial**.
- **Interventional therapy**: After the trial period, the patient reports significant pain reduction and is offered a **spinal cord stimulator implantation** for long-term relief.

**Outcome**: After 6 months, the patient reports a substantial decrease in pain intensity and an improvement in functionality, allowing him to return to daily activities with minimal opioid use.

**Discussion**: This case illustrates the importance of an integrated, **multidisciplinary approach** to managing chronic low back pain, combining pharmacological interventions, interventional techniques, and physical and psychological therapies.

## Case Study 3: Neuropathic Pain Following Stroke

**Patient**: A 72-year-old woman with post-stroke neuropathic pain.

**Clinical Scenario**: The patient has been living with partial paralysis following a stroke 6 months ago.
She presents with a complaint of **burning, stabbing pain** in her right arm, which has progressively worsened and is not relieved by standard analgesics.

**Assessment and Management**:
- **Diagnosis**: The clinical presentation, along with MRI findings of a **cerebrovascular event** in the somatosensory cortex, suggests **central post-stroke pain (CPSP)**, a form of neuropathic pain.
- **Pharmacologic treatment**: Initially, **gabapentin** is prescribed, with a slow titration to achieve the therapeutic dose. When this does not fully control the pain, **tricyclic antidepressants** (amitriptyline) are added to the regimen.
- **Interventional approach**: A **selective nerve block** and **transcranial magnetic stimulation (TMS)** are considered to help modulate pain perception in the affected area of the brain.

**Outcome**: The patient's pain reduces by 50%, allowing for improved functional abilities and a decreased reliance on opioids.

**Discussion**: Managing **neuropathic pain** after a

stroke requires both a solid understanding of the pathophysiology of CPSP and a combination of pharmacological, interventional, and psychological approaches to improve quality of life.

## Case Study 4: Fibromyalgia Management

**Patient**: A 45-year-old woman diagnosed with fibromyalgia.

**Clinical Scenario**: The patient reports widespread musculoskeletal pain, fatigue, and sleep disturbances.

Her pain is exacerbated by stress, and she has been unable to find relief with standard analgesics.

**Assessment and Management**:

- **Comprehensive evaluation**: A **pain diary** is kept to identify triggers, and **blood tests** are used to rule out other causes of widespread pain.
- **Pharmacological treatment**: Duloxetine (an SNRI) is started to address both pain and associated depressive symptoms. **Pregabalin** is added for its effectiveness in neuropathic pain.
- **Non-pharmacological treatment**: Cognitive Behavioral Therapy (CBT) is initiated to help the patient develop better coping strategies for dealing with pain and stress. A **graded exercise program** is also implemented to improve physical functioning.

**Outcome**: Over a 6-month period, the patient reports a significant reduction in pain levels, improved sleep quality, and a better sense of emotional well-being. She is able to return to part-time work and engage in regular physical activity.

**Discussion**: Fibromyalgia requires a **holistic management approach**, focusing not just on pain relief, but also on improving sleep, reducing fatigue, and addressing emotional well-being.

## Case Study 5: Cancer Pain Management

**Patient**: A 58-year-old male with advanced prostate cancer.

**Clinical Scenario**: The patient presents with **bone pain** in the pelvis, associated with **advanced metastatic prostate cancer**. Despite being on opioids, his pain remains poorly controlled, and he experiences significant side effects.

**Assessment and Management**:
- **Pain assessment**: The patient's pain is assessed using the **McGill Pain Questionnaire**, revealing a mixed pattern of somatic and neuropathic pain.
- **Multimodal approach**: The oncology team initiates **radiotherapy** to target the metastatic bone lesions. Additionally, **bisphosphonates** (zoledronic acid) are given to help manage pain and prevent further bone degradation.
- **Opioid rotation**: Given his opioid intolerance, the patient is transitioned to **fentanyl patches** for more consistent pain control.
- **Palliative care**: A palliative care specialist is involved to manage the patient's pain in the context of end-stage disease, providing holistic support and symptom management.

**Outcome**: After initiating radiation therapy and adjusting the pain medications, the patient reports a significant reduction in pain and better overall quality of life, allowing him to spend more time with family.

**Discussion**: Effective **cancer pain management** requires a team-based approach, addressing both the **physical** and **psychosocial** aspects of care. **Palliative care** plays an essential role in improving the patient's comfort during advanced illness.

## Case Study 6: Acute Herpetic Neuralgia

**Patient**: A 55-year-old male with herpes zoster (shingles).

**Clinical Scenario**: The patient presents with a painful rash on his left chest, diagnosed as **herpes zoster**.

After a course of antiviral medication, he continues to experience burning pain in the affected area, even though the rash has healed.

His pain is described as **sharp, burning, and persistent**, and he rates it as 7/10 on the pain scale.

**Assessment and Management**:
- **Diagnosis**: The patient's ongoing pain is diagnosed as **post-herpetic neuralgia (PHN)**, a common complication of shingles.
- **Pharmacological treatment**: Initial treatment with **gabapentin** and **lidocaine patches** is initiated to help manage the neuropathic pain. The patient is also given a **topical capsaicin cream** to reduce pain.
- **Psychosocial support**: Given the chronic nature of the pain, **cognitive behavioral therapy (CBT)** is suggested

to help with pain coping mechanisms.

**Outcome**: After 3 months, the patient reports a reduction in pain by 50%, with a significant improvement in quality of life and functionality. The combination of oral medications, topical agents, and CBT proves effective.

**Discussion**: **Post-herpetic neuralgia** can be difficult to manage. This case demonstrates the **importance of early intervention** with both pharmacological treatments and

non-pharmacological strategies to prevent long-term pain.

## Case Study 7: Pain Management In A Patient With Rheumatoid Arthritis

**Patient**: A 60-year-old woman with rheumatoid arthritis (RA).

**Clinical Scenario**: The patient with longstanding rheumatoid arthritis presents with **exacerbation of joint pain** in the wrists, knees, and shoulders.

Her current treatment regimen includes **methotrexate** and **hydroxychloroquine**, but she reports that pain and stiffness have increased despite these medications.

**Assessment and Management**:
- **Diagnosis**: The patient's exacerbation is assessed with an **imaging study** (X-rays) revealing significant **joint damage** and **inflammation**.
- **Pharmacological treatment**: She is started on a **biologic agent** (etanercept) to target the underlying disease activity and is prescribed **NSAIDs** for symptomatic relief.
- **Non-pharmacological treatment**: Physical therapy and

**heat/cold therapy** are added to the treatment plan to reduce stiffness and improve joint mobility.

**Outcome**: After 6 weeks, the patient reports a 40% reduction in pain levels, improved joint movement, and fewer episodes of stiffness. She feels more mobile and can perform daily tasks with less discomfort.

**Discussion**: In **rheumatoid arthritis**, managing the underlying inflammation with **disease-modifying anti-rheumatic drugs (DMARDs)** is essential for long-term pain control. Combining pharmacological treatments with **physical therapy** can improve both pain and function.

## Case Study 8: Cancer-Related Pain In A Palliative Care Setting

**Patient**: A 70-year-old male with terminal lung cancer.

**Clinical Scenario**: The patient, diagnosed with **advanced non-small cell lung cancer**, is in hospice care and presents with **severe, diffuse pain** due to metastatic disease involving the lungs, liver, and bones.

He is experiencing pain despite being on opioid therapy, including **morphine** for breakthrough pain.

**Assessment and Management**:
- **Pain assessment**: The pain is assessed using the **McGill Pain Questionnaire**, revealing a mix of **somatic and visceral pain**.
- **Pharmacological approach**: The opioid dosage is increased, and a **fentanyl patch** is applied for

continuous release. **Adjuvant medications**, such as **steroids** for inflammation and **bisphosphonates** for bone pain, are introduced.

- **Palliative care**: A focus on **comfort care** is implemented, with additional psychological support to manage the patient's anxiety and existential distress.

**Outcome**: After adjustment to the pain regimen, the patient reports a significant decrease in pain intensity, allowing him to spend quality time with family and reducing his distress.

**Discussion**: Managing **cancer-related pain** involves a **holistic approach** that combines pharmacologic interventions with psychosocial support. **Palliative care** is key to enhancing comfort and quality of life, even in the end stages of disease.

## Case Study 9: Pain Management In A Patient With Complex Regional Pain Syndrome (Crps)

**Patient**: A 30-year-old female with complex regional pain syndrome (CRPS) following a wrist fracture.

**Clinical Scenario**: The patient reports **severe, burning pain** in her right wrist and forearm, following a distal radius fracture that occurred 6 months ago.

Despite healing of the fracture, the pain persists and has become disabling.

The pain is associated with **swelling, changes in skin color, and sensitivity to touch**.

**Assessment and Management**:

- **Diagnosis**: The diagnosis of **CRPS** is made based on clinical examination and **sympathetic nerve block** (which temporarily relieves the pain).
- **Pharmacological treatment**: The patient is started on **gabapentin** for neuropathic pain and **NSAIDs** for inflammation.
- **Interventional therapy**: After a trial of **nerve blocks**, the patient is referred for a **spinal cord stimulation** evaluation, as pharmacologic treatments alone are insufficient.
- **Psychosocial therapy**: **CBT** is initiated to address her **depression** and **anxiety**, which are contributing to the pain experience.

**Outcome**: The patient experiences a significant reduction in pain after starting spinal cord stimulation and continues to improve with psychological support.

**Discussion**: **CRPS** is a challenging condition that requires a **multidisciplinary approach** involving pharmacological therapy, interventional procedures, and psychological support to manage both the physical and emotional aspects of the disorder.

## Case Study 10: Acute Abdominal Pain In A Patient With Gallbladder Disease

**Patient**: A 45-year-old male with acute gallbladder disease.

**Clinical Scenario**: The patient presents with **severe right upper quadrant abdominal pain**, associated with nausea and vomiting. He has a history of **intermittent biliary colic** over the past year, and ultrasound reveals **gallstones** and signs of **acute**

cholecystitis.

**Assessment and Management**:

- **Diagnosis**: The diagnosis of **acute cholecystitis** is confirmed with imaging and clinical findings.
- **Pain management**: The patient is given **IV opioids** (hydromorphone) for acute pain relief. Once stabilized, **NSAIDs** (ketorolac) are added to address both pain and inflammation.
- **Surgical intervention**: The patient is referred for **laparoscopic cholecystectomy** once the acute inflammation is under control.

**Outcome**: The patient's pain resolves postoperatively after the gallbladder is removed, and he is discharged with oral **NSAIDs** for pain management and instructions for postoperative care.

**Discussion**: Acute abdominal pain due to **gallbladder disease** requires timely **pain management** and **surgical intervention**. **Opioids** are effective for short-term pain control, but NSAIDs can be introduced for their anti-inflammatory effects once the patient is stable.

## Case Study 11: Diabetic Neuropathy

**Patient**: A 62-year-old male with type 2 diabetes.

**Clinical Scenario**: The patient presents with **numbness, tingling**, and **burning sensations** in his feet, which have been worsening over the past 6 months.

His blood glucose levels have been poorly controlled, with an HbA1c of 9.5%.

He also reports difficulty walking due to foot pain.

**Assessment and Management**:
- **Diagnosis**: **Diabetic peripheral neuropathy** (DPN) is diagnosed based on clinical symptoms, a **positive monofilament test**, and reduced sensation on the feet.
- **Pharmacological treatment**: **Gabapentin** is started to manage neuropathic pain, with **duloxetine** added as an adjuvant for pain and potential depressive symptoms.
- **Lifestyle modification**: The patient is referred to a **diabetes educator** for better glucose control and foot care.
- **Psychosocial support**: **CBT** is recommended to help manage his stress and frustration with his condition.

**Outcome**: After 8 weeks, the patient reports a 50% reduction in pain, improved mobility, and better control over his blood glucose levels.

**Discussion**: **Diabetic neuropathy** requires a comprehensive treatment approach, including **glucose control**, **pharmacologic pain management**, and **foot care** to prevent progression of the condition.

## Case Study 12: Low Back Pain

**Patient**: A 45-year-old female with acute low back pain.

**Clinical Scenario**: The patient presents with **acute low back pain** following a heavy lifting incident at work.

She describes the pain as **sharp, localized to the lower back**, and rates it as 8/10.

She denies any radiation of pain to the legs but reports significant stiffness.

**Assessment and Management:**
- **Diagnosis**: Acute **musculoskeletal low back pain**, likely due to muscle strain, is diagnosed based on the clinical history and physical examination.
- **Pharmacological treatment**: The patient is prescribed **NSAIDs** (ibuprofen) for pain relief and advised to use **heat therapy** for muscle relaxation.
- **Non-pharmacological treatment**: **Physical therapy** is recommended to improve strength and flexibility, with a focus on posture and lifting techniques.

**Outcome**: The patient experiences significant improvement in pain within 2 weeks and is able to return to work with modified duties.

**Discussion**: Acute **low back pain** is a common issue that can often be treated conservatively with **NSAIDs** and **physical therapy**, avoiding the need for imaging unless red flags are present.

## Case Study 13: Pain Management In Sickle Cell Disease

**Patient**: A 25-year-old female with sickle cell disease.

**Clinical Scenario**: The patient presents with a **pain crisis** characterized by severe, throbbing pain in the chest, back, and legs, which she rates as 9/10.

She has a history of frequent pain crises, requiring hospitalization for pain management in the past.

**Assessment and Management:**
- **Diagnosis: Sickle cell pain crisis** is diagnosed based on

her history and clinical presentation.
- **Pharmacological treatment**: The patient is started on **IV opioids** (morphine) for acute pain relief. **Hydration** and **oxygen therapy** are also initiated to help alleviate sickling and reduce pain.
- **Adjuvant therapy**: **Hydroxyurea** is discussed as a long-term therapy to reduce the frequency of pain crises.
- **Psychosocial support**: The patient is referred to a **pain management specialist** for ongoing care and coping strategies.

**Outcome**: The patient's pain improves after a few days of hospitalization, and she is discharged with **oral opioids** for home management and a plan for follow-up care.

**Discussion**: **Sickle cell disease** requires a multidisciplinary approach to pain management, balancing **acute opioid treatment** with **long-term strategies** to reduce crisis frequency and improve quality of life.

## Case Study 14: Postoperative Pain Management

**Patient**: A 68-year-old male who underwent total knee arthroplasty (TKA).

**Clinical Scenario**: The patient is recovering from **total knee replacement surgery** and reports **moderate pain** in the knee joint postoperatively.
The pain is sharp and localized, and the patient is experiencing difficulty moving the knee.

**Assessment and Management**:

- **Diagnosis**: **Postoperative pain** following knee arthroplasty.
- **Pharmacological treatment**: The patient is prescribed **opioids** (oxycodone) for acute pain relief and **NSAIDs** (celecoxib) for inflammation control.
- **Non-pharmacological treatment**: The patient is enrolled in **physical therapy** to encourage early mobilization, which is crucial for recovery.
- **Interventional therapy**: A **continuous femoral nerve block** is used postoperatively to help manage pain and reduce opioid requirements.

**Outcome**: The patient has a smooth recovery, with significant improvement in mobility and pain reduction after 2 weeks.

**Discussion**: Effective **postoperative pain management** after knee surgery involves a **multimodal approach**, including both pharmacological and non-pharmacological treatments to facilitate recovery and minimize opioid use.

## Case Study 15: Trigeminal Neuralgia

**Patient**: A 57-year-old female with trigeminal neuralgia.

**Clinical Scenario**: The patient presents with **sharp, stabbing facial pain** on the right side of her face, particularly around the cheek and jaw, triggered by mild touch, such as brushing her teeth.

The pain lasts for seconds to minutes and is excruciating, rating it 9/10.

**Assessment and Management:**
- **Diagnosis: Trigeminal neuralgia** is diagnosed based on the classic pain pattern and physical examination.
- **Pharmacological treatment**: The patient is started on **carbamazepine**, which is considered first-line treatment for trigeminal neuralgia.
- **Surgical option**: If pharmacological therapy does not provide relief, **microvascular decompression** or **gamma knife radiosurgery** is considered as a potential treatment.

**Outcome**: The patient reports complete resolution of the pain after starting carbamazepine, with no side effects after a few weeks of treatment.

**Discussion: Trigeminal neuralgia** is a classic example of **neurovascular pain** and often responds well to **carbamazepine**. Surgical intervention can be considered in refractory cases.

## Case Study 16: Cluster Headache

**Patient**: A 34-year-old male with a history of cluster headaches.

**Clinical Scenario**: The patient presents with **unilateral, severe periorbital pain**, associated with **lacrimation, rhinorrhea**, and restlessness.
The pain episodes occur daily, each lasting 45 minutes to 2 hours, and have been ongoing for the past week.

**Assessment and Management:**
- **Diagnosis: Cluster headache** is diagnosed based on the

patient's history and characteristic symptoms.
- **Acute treatment**: The patient is treated with **100% oxygen therapy** (for acute attacks) and prescribed **sumatriptan injections** for immediate relief.
- **Preventive treatment**: **Verapamil** is started as a preventive measure to reduce the frequency of attacks.

**Outcome**: After 2 weeks, the patient experiences a reduction in the frequency and severity of the attacks, with minimal side effects from treatment.

**Discussion**: **Cluster headaches** require **aggressive treatment** during acute attacks, such as **oxygen therapy** and **triptans**, with **verapamil** used for prevention.

## Case Study 17: Chronic Migraines

**Patient**: A 42-year-old female with chronic migraines.

**Clinical Scenario**: The patient presents with a history of **recurrent, throbbing headaches** for the past 5 years.

She reports having headaches at least 15 days per month, often associated with **nausea, light sensitivity**, and **aura**. She rates the pain as 7/10 during an attack.

**Assessment and Management**:
- **Diagnosis**: **Chronic migraine** is diagnosed based on the frequency and nature of the headaches.
- **Pharmacological treatment**: The patient is started on **propranolol** for migraine prevention, and **triptans** are prescribed for acute attacks.
- **Behavioral interventions**: **Cognitive behavioral therapy (CBT)** is recommended to help the patient cope

with stress and manage triggers.

**Outcome**: After 3 months, the patient reports a reduction in headache frequency and severity, with a 40% decrease in the number of headache days per month.

**Discussion**: Chronic migraine management requires a **multifaceted approach** including **preventive medication**, **acute treatments**, and **lifestyle modifications**.

## Case Study 18: Post-Surgical Pain Following Abdominal Hysterectomy

**Patient**: A 49-year-old female who underwent abdominal hysterectomy.

**Clinical Scenario**: The patient is recovering from **abdominal hysterectomy** and presents with **moderate to severe pain** in the abdominal area, particularly when moving or coughing. She rates her pain as 6/10.

**Assessment and Management**:
- **Diagnosis**: **Postoperative pain** following abdominal surgery.
- **Pharmacological treatment**: The patient is started on **IV opioids** (morphine) for pain relief, which is later transitioned to **oral opioids**.
- **Non-pharmacological treatment**: **Deep breathing exercises** and **mobilization** are encouraged to improve circulation and decrease the risk of complications like DVT.
- **Interventional therapy**: A **nerve block** is considered

if pain is not well controlled with pharmacologic treatments.

**Outcome**: The patient shows gradual improvement in pain and mobility, with eventual discontinuation of opioid therapy after 1 week.

**Discussion**: Postoperative pain management after **abdominal surgery** involves a **multimodal approach**, balancing **opioid therapy** with non-pharmacological interventions to reduce the need for pain medication.

## Case Study 19: Fibromyalgia

**Patient**: A 38-year-old female with widespread pain.

**Clinical Scenario**: The patient presents with a 2-year history of **widespread musculoskeletal pain**, fatigue, and **poor sleep**.

She reports difficulty concentrating and feels "exhausted" even after a full night's sleep.

She is also experiencing **tender points** in the neck, shoulders, and lower back.

**Assessment and Management**:
- **Diagnosis**: **Fibromyalgia** is diagnosed based on clinical symptoms and the presence of **tender points**.
- **Pharmacological treatment**: The patient is started on **duloxetine** for both pain and mood support. **Pregabalin** is considered for pain management.
- **Non-pharmacological treatment**: The patient is referred to **cognitive behavioral therapy** (CBT) and a **physical therapist** to improve function and manage symptoms.

**Outcome**: After 6 weeks, the patient reports significant improvements in pain and fatigue, with better sleep and functioning.

**Discussion**: **Fibromyalgia** requires **multidisciplinary management**, combining **medication** for pain and mood, along with **CBT** and **exercise** to improve overall function and quality of life.

## Case Study 20: Complex Regional Pain Syndrome (Crps)

**Patient**: A 48-year-old male post-trauma.

**Clinical Scenario**: The patient presents with **persistent, severe pain** and **swelling** in his right wrist following a **distal radius fracture** 6 weeks ago. His symptoms include **skin color changes, temperature differences**, and **sensitivity to touch** in the affected area.

**Assessment and Management**:
- **Diagnosis**: **Complex regional pain syndrome (CRPS)** is suspected based on the clinical presentation.
- **Pharmacological treatment**: The patient is started on **gabapentin** for neuropathic pain, with a trial of **bisphosphonates** to reduce bone resorption.
- **Physical therapy**: The patient is referred for **desensitization exercises** and **gradual mobilization**.
- **Psychological support**: **CBT** is recommended to address the patient's anxiety and depression due to chronic pain.

**Outcome**: The patient experiences significant improvement in pain and mobility after 3 months of treatment.

**Discussion**: **CRPS** management involves a **multidisciplinary approach** with **medication**, **physical therapy**, and **psychosocial support** for optimal outcomes.

# ABOUT THE AUTHOR

**Dr Essam Abdelhakim**

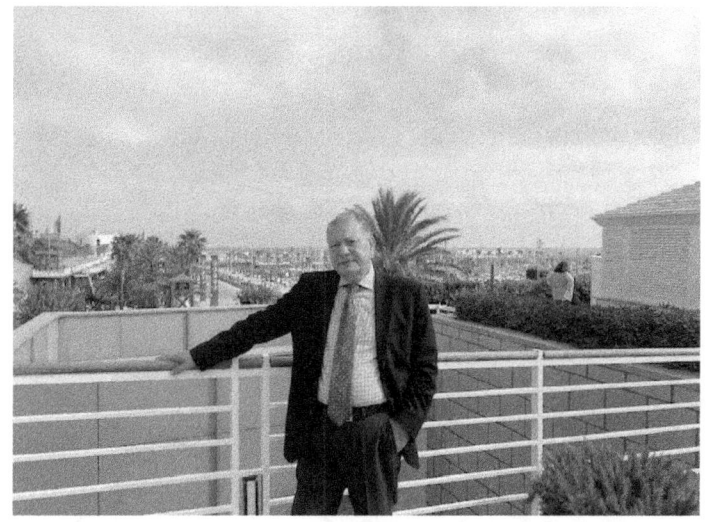

Senior Consultant and Expert in Medical Education

# DISCLOSURE

**Disclosure**

This book has been created with the assistance of *Artificial Intelligence (AI) tools* and thoroughly reviewed and edited by the author to ensure clarity, relevance, and educational value.

While every effort has been made to provide accurate and up-to-date information, this content is intended solely for educational and informational purposes.

The author is a medical professional; however, the information provided in this book *is not a substitute for professional medical advice, diagnosis, or treatment.*

**Readers are strongly advised** to consult licensed healthcare providers or specialists for any medical concerns or conditions.

By using this book, **you acknowledge and agree** that the author shall not be held responsible or liable for any loss, damage, or harm whether physical, emotional, financial, or otherwise that may occur *as a result of the use or misuse of the information presented herein.*

www.ingramcontent.com/pod-product-compliance
Lightning Source LLC
Chambersburg PA
CBHW070115230526
45472CB00004B/1262